Th

True Sexual Weirdness
from the World's News

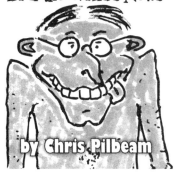

by Chris Pilbeam

Crombie Jardine
PUBLISHING LIMITED

13 Nonsuch Walk, Cheam, Surrey, SM2 7LG
www.crombiejardine.com

Published by Crombie Jardine Publishing Limited
First edition, 2005

ISBN 1-905102-38-0

Written by Chris Pilbeam
Cover illustration by Bobb Gibbs
Designed by www.glensaville.com
Printed & bound in the United Kingdom by
William Clowes Ltd, Beccles, Suffolk

CONTENTS

INTRODUCTION 7

PEEPING TOM TAKES A TUMBLE 10

THE EDINBURGH CONE-HUMPER 12

FAMILY DOG BECOMES NEW
BRIDE'S LOVE RIVAL 15

DRIVE-BY PORNOGRAPHY 18

PERVERT LIKES HIS VEGETABLES 20

HOW NOT TO GET YOUR FIRST GIRLFRIEND . . . 23

'REALISTIC' SEX DOLL SPARKS
MURDER INVESTIGATION 26

STAR WARS FAN TAKES IT TOO FAR 28

GOAT LOVER RUINS TRAIN RIDE
FOR EVERYBODY 31

SEX GHOST TERRORISES ISLAND 35

FLASHER LEARNS THE HARD WAY. 37

ATTACK OF THE FOOT-LICKER. 40

MAN'S CHOICE OF SWIMWEAR
FAILS TO IMPRESS .42

THE NAKED PHOTOGRAPHER 44

COWS JOIN THE FIGHT
AGAINST SEX IN PUBLIC 45

MOTORWAY SEX UNEARTHS LEGAL LOOPHOLE . . .47

NAKED PEEPER ON THE LOOSE. 49

SUSPECT PACKAGE BLOWS UP. 52

THE WORST TRAINSPOTTER EVER. 54

DUTCHMAN TAKES THE P*SS 57

DUCK DOESN'T TAKE NO FOR AN ANSWER 59

JAPANESE GROPERS FIND
STRENGTH IN NUMBERS 61

FLASH PHOTOGRAPHY 64

GOAT MAN UNSURPRISINGLY 'EMBARRASSED' . 66

MAN GETS LUCKY WITH PIG 68

AMERICA'S WORST-DRESSED CRIMINAL 69

THE DANGEROUS WORLD OF PANTY FETISHES . . 72

CHINA/JAPAN RELATIONS
NOT HELPED BY ORGY 74

BRIDEGROOM'S HAPPINESS DEFLATED 76

NO LAWYER IS THIS IMPRESSIVE 78

SHOE HOARDER ONLY LIKES LEFT FEET 80

PERV ARMED ROBBER ISN'T GREEDY 82

TRAFFIC CAMERA WANTS TO LIVE A LITTLE . . . 83

AFGHAN SOLDIER MAKES AN ASS OF HIMSELF . . 85

THE HAIRCUT BANDIT 87

A MAN IS A DOG'S WORST FRIEND 90

PROBABLY THE BEST BOSS IN THE WORLD . . . 92

PORN LIVENS UP A DULL DAY IN PARLIAMENT . . 94

MEDICAL FETISHIST BANNED
FROM HOSPITALS. 95

PORN NOW SAFE FOR THE RELIGIOUS 98

EX-COP NO LONGER TAKES PIG JOKES WELL . . 100

DIY SURGEON'S CAREER SNIPPED SHORT . . . 102

NAKED DOG-WRESTLING WOMAN
'DOES IT ALL THE TIME'. 105

KIDNAP FANTASY FAILS TO AMUSE POLICE . . 108

THIS IS CLUCKED UP 111

IN CONCLUSION... I SAT ON IT BY
ACCIDENT, HONEST 117

INTRODUCTION

A tourist walks into a country pub, where an old man is sitting sadly at the bar.

"I built this pub," said the old man to the tourist. "But do they call me Fred the builder? No, they don't."

"I planted that beautiful garden outside," the old man continues. "And do they call me Fred the gardener? No, they don't."

"I even made the chairs we're sitting on," says the old man, his voice rising. "Do they call me Fred the carpenter? No, they don't."

"But I shag just *one* chicken..."

This is a dossier of truly bizarre sexual misbehaviour from around the world. Some of these people, like the old man, shagged just one chicken. Some of them chose a dog instead. One of them chose

a traffic cone on a busy street.
One of them took his blow-up doll
to meet his parents. One of them
has a thing for waist-length
hair. One of them has a thing
for surgical masks. One of them
has a thing for falling through
bathroom ceilings while spying on
people. One of them has a thing
for exposing himself to traffic
with a cucumber in his mouth...

Weird?

There's much, much more.

PEEPING TOM TAKES A TUMBLE

A Canadian peeping tom who crawled into ceilings to spy on women was caught when he crashed through the ceiling of the ladies' bathroom in a DIY store.

Stewart Charles Ryan, 28, had clambered into the tiled ceiling of the adjacent men's bathroom and crawled through the roof space to get an eyeful of the female customers. All was going to plan until Ryan's flimsy perch gave out from under him, leaving him in a compromising situation on the floor below. Ryan managed to flee, but had been caught on camera and was swiftly picked up and forced to explain himself.

THE EDINBURGH CONE-HUMPER

"I was disgusted and embarrassed," said one witness to the Scottish capital of Edinburgh's worst piece of street theatre ever – 34-year-old Ross Watt's public simulation of sex with a traffic cone in a busy street.

Watt, who already had a previous conviction for simulating sex with a training shoe in a public place, spent most of the afternoon in question approaching groups of teenagers in the city and asking to buy their trainers. When he eventually failed to get his hands on a pair, he decided instead to give passers-by a 'public show' with a traffic cone. In a display that lasted an impressive 20 minutes, startled onlookers were treated to the sight of Watt humping the cone in the street, encircled by cars full of teenagers screaming at him to 'give it some'.

Watt escaped jail with a stern warning from a judge not to repeat his 'disgusting behaviour' again – despite having already been on probation for 'hitting himself repeatedly in the groin with a training shoe while standing in the window of his flat'.

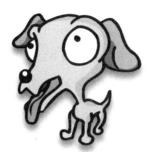

FAMILY DOG BECOMES NEW BRIDE'S LOVE RIVAL

A woman catching her new
husband having sex with the
family dog is bad. When the
husband tells her that he's in
love with the dog and wants

a divorce, it's really bad.

This was the fate of a 20-year-old Cambodian woman who came home to her house in the capital, Phnom Penh, to find her 24-year-old husband in a 'passionate embrace' with their dog. The husband proclaimed his undying love for the animal and the woman called police – only to have them tell her that there was nothing they could do about it.

"The husband told us, yes, of

course he did it," said the local chief of police. "But we could only solve the problem of them wanting a divorce. Under Cambodian law, the relationship with his dog is not strictly illegal."

Police later said that the man had moved back in with his mother. Sadly, they gave nothing away as to the whereabouts of the dog.

DRIVE-BY PORNOGRAPHY

If you're going to play pornography on your car's onboard DVD player, don't drive slowly past a police station while you're doing it. Cops in New York recently busted 35-year-old Andre Gainey for driving around town with X-rated movie 'Chocolate Foam' clearly on display through the windows of his car.

"The windows weren't tinted at all," fumed a police spokesman. "It could have been seen by a family that was parked behind him." The inconsiderate Gainey was sentenced to spend the next three weekends in jail for his little display.

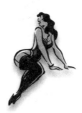

PERVERT LIKES HIS VEGETABLES

'A fat man in women's clothes with a cucumber in his mouth is exposing himself to traffic on the main road,' is not something a policeman wants to hear.

Hard luck, then, for officers in Moss – a little Norwegian town where the local police rarely have to deal with anything worse than a stray elk on the road. They heard the sentence

in a call from a worried
motorist one night in 2004.

We can only guess at what else
the flasher was doing - when
asked to give more details, the
motorist reporting him refused
on the grounds that he was in
a car with children and didn't
want them to hear him say it.

A patrol car sped off to the
stretch of the road, but the
man had vanished. He appeared
again later, treating several

more drivers to the same sight,
but then vanished, never to
be seen again. A disappointed
police spokesman confessed to
reporters that the significance
of the cucumber would have
to remain a mystery.

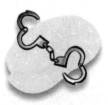

HOW NOT TO GET YOUR FIRST GIRLFRIEND

A group of South African teenagers are setting a new low for adolescent behaviour by masturbating en masse in the street. The town of Tzaneen has been plagued by incidents of public masturbation – accompanied by joyful screaming – since the beginning of 2005.

"One of them just held up his

penis for everyone to see and started masturbating," said Gloria Shingange, who had walked past the group while wearing a miniskirt. "He then closed his eyes, grimaced and shouted at the top of his voice in apparent enjoyment of what he was doing. I was somewhat embarrassed."

Unlike most teenagers, who would rather die than discuss the subject, one of the culprits was perfectly happy to give his side of the story.

"I feel very happy after relieving my sexual appetite by masturbating near to a woman with beautiful legs," the lad said. "After all, there is no girl out there who wants a filthy glue-sniffing street kid."

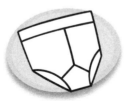

'REALISTIC' SEX DOLL SPARKS MURDER INVESTIGATION

A German man became the suspect of a murder investigation after he purchased an 'ultra-realistic' sex doll and took it home. A terrified neighbour called police and reported that a man was dragging a dead body up the stairs outside her flat, and the cops swung into action.

The murder suspect was

apparently 'surprised and disturbed' to be confronted by officers at his door, but was only too happy to invite them inside and show them his new purchase, which he had been in the middle of 'deflowering' when he was disturbed. He also treated the cops to a guided tour of the four other sex dolls in his collection, at which point they decided to leave the non-murderer alone as soon as possible.

STAR WARS FAN TAKES IT TOO FAR

"At first, I thought he was a die-hard *Star Wars* fan trying to impress us with his costume," said a Malaysian woman of her recent odd experience with a man in full Darth Vader regalia. "We were most shocked when he showed us his privates."

The woman and several of her friends were waiting at a bus stop in the town of

Baru Nilai when the Darth Vader impersonator emerged from a nearby car. According to witnesses, he 'strutted about menacingly', then whipped out his genitals.

When the women screamed, the man leapt back into his car and sped off. His identity remains a mystery and locals have vowed to be on their guard in future.

"Next time," said another witness, "it will not be 'Revenge of the

Sith' but revenge on a sick man if
we catch him doing his act again."

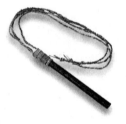

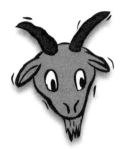

GOAT LOVER RUINS TRAIN RIDE FOR EVERYBODY

You can expect to see many interesting sights on a train journey through the English countryside, but only rarely will you see a 23-year-old

chef, pants around ankles,
having sex with a goat.

Stephen Hall might have got away
with his romantic escapade if
the Hull to Bridlington express,
with dozens of people on board,
hadn't stopped at signals next
to the allotments he'd found
the goat in. Police switchboards
jammed within seconds as the
train's passengers reported him
en masse. Cops raced to the
scene to find that two passers-
by had already apprehended Hall

and freed the goat, which Hall had romantically lassoed and tethered to a shed with his belt.

"I have never done anything like this before," Hall later told the media after pleading guilty to a charge of buggery. "My friends have been giving me a lot of stick. They are all joking with me about it."

The goat, meanwhile, was said to be 'subdued' after its brief courtship.

"It didn't seem too upset,"
said a police spokesman,
"but it is difficult to tell."

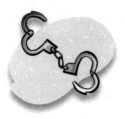

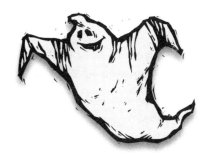

SEX GHOST TERRORISES ISLAND

Residents of the African island of Zanzibar are very upset about the antics of a homosexual ghost called Popo Bawa who apparently turns up in men's houses in the

night and has his way with them –
but only during general elections.

According to his 'victims', Popo
Bawa's presence is apparently
revealed by a puff of smoke,
after which he puts men in
a trance and forces them to
submit to his hot ghost love.
No one knows why he only
comes out during general
elections. He just does.

He also seems to have a sense
of humour – victims say that

he threatens to come back
the next night unless they
tell all their friends what
just happened to them.

FLASHER LEARNS
THE HARD WAY

If there were a handbook for
flashers, the first rule would
be not to expose oneself to
people with large, fierce dogs.
However, there is no handbook

- so a Croatian flasher had
to learn the hard way.

Witnesses said that the 36-year-
old man was visibly drunk when
he staggered up to a garden
fence in front of a woman's
house in Zagreb and pushed
his genitals through a hole in
it. It obviously never occurred
to him that the woman's dog
might be in the garden. The dog
bounded up to the fence and
sank its teeth into his privates,
leaving the man attached to

the fence, howling in agony.

The flasher managed to free himself but, due to the 'serious injuries' he suffered in escaping, didn't get far before being picked up by the cops. After a painful ride to hospital in a police car, the now-sober exhibitionist was fined for violating public order and 'insulting the moral feelings of citizens'.

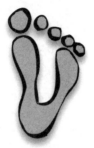

ATTACK OF THE FOOT-LICKER

An American woman was 'extremely annoyed' after becoming the latest victim of Raymond Dublin, foot-licker extraordinaire, a court heard recently.

36-year-old Dublin pleaded guilty to creeping up behind the woman in the 'Save-A-Lot' supermarket in the town of Bellingham, Massachusetts, dropping to his knees and licking her feet. The woman's irritation was compounded by the fact that this was her third encounter with the foot-licker, who had just served a one-year sentence for doing exactly the same thing to someone else in another supermarket.

MAN'S CHOICE OF SWIMWEAR FAILS TO IMPRESS

On June 8th, 2004, a police officer received a number of complaints about an inappropriately dressed man on Eastbourne's Holywell beach. Investigating, the officer was treated to the horrific sight of 60-year-old Richard Stofer reclining in the sun, entirely naked and with a pair of ladies' underwear next to him.

Stofer was given a stern warning

to cover up, but reappeared a week later on a different beach, this time in 'transparent ladies' underwear'. A week after that, style-conscious Stofer came to the attention of police again, this time for wearing a 'small, heart-shaped ladies' thong' which 'clearly exposed his genitalia'.

A judge has now threatened Stofer with five years in jail if he is caught 'publicly parading naked anywhere in the county of Sussex other than a nudist beach'.

THE NAKED PHOTOGRAPHER

Police in the American town of Columbus, Ohio, are hunting an amateur photographer with an irritating habit.

The 'Naked Photographer' has so far struck 37 times. He does his work entirely in the nude, apart from a baseball cap and sunglasses. His technique is to leap out at women, photograph their expressions, and then vanish.

Despite female officers patrolling the streets in plain clothes for over a year in the hope of catching him, the nude lensman remains at large.

COWS JOIN THE FIGHT AGAINST SEX IN PUBLIC

A small Dutch town has released Highland cattle into its parks to prevent couples having sex in them. Fed up with outdoor-

sex enthusiasts upsetting
his citizens, the mayor of
Spaarnwoude decided to buy the
huge animals in the hope that
they will scare the offenders off.

The idea isn't without precedent
- cases of open-air love at
a nature reserve elsewhere
in Holland have apparently
dropped dramatically after the
authorities released several
Highland cattle into their grounds.

"Lets face it," said a park

ranger, "having a two-ton hairy beast with huge horns looking at you isn't exactly going to put you in the mood for love."

MOTORWAY SEX UNEARTHS LEGAL LOOPHOLE

In Germany, it's not illegal to have sex while driving on the motorway.

We know this because a Cologne man who took out a road sign

at 60mph while having sex
with a blonde hitchhiker he'd
just picked up was only fined
£400 for fleeing the scene
of the accident – with the
naked hitchhiker in tow.

"It's a situation lawmakers never
thought about," a spokesman
for Cologne magistrates court
admitted after the case.

NAKED PEEPER ON THE LOOSE

"The residents of Malvani village have complained to us about one man who comes and troubles them late at night," a police officer from the Indian state of Maharashtra told journalists recently. "We are keeping a vigil around the village, but we cannot locate him."

It's not a vampire: it's the nude peeping tom of Malvani. Villagers say that he creeps into the village only between 1am and 2am, where he stands naked in front of open windows until he's spotted, at which point he flees at lightning speed.

Resident Eugenia D'Souza described being disturbed by strange noises in the night. When she tried to see what the noise was, she was treated to the unpleasant sight of a naked man trying to climb up the frame of the window she was looking out of. When she screamed, he bolted.

"He is so quick that none of us can catch him," said D'Souza. "The only article that we've found has been a slipper at the gate. All we know is that he is tall, fair and has curly hair."

"The man was not wearing anything," said resident Anjali Machado of her own encounter with the mystery man. "Since he didn't try to steal anything, he definitely couldn't have been a robber. He is obviously a pervert."

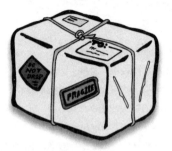

SUSPECT PACKAGE BLOWS UP

A suspect package that began buzzing in a Berlin post office turned out to be a sex doll with a faulty starter switch.

Panicking postal workers called

the bomb squad when the package began vibrating and making strange noises. Officers picked up the man who had sent the package and brought him to the post office to see if he could shed some light on the matter.

The embarrassed sender had to explain to all present that the 'bomb' was actually a vibrating blow-up sex doll that he was returning to the manufacturers because it kept switching itself on unexpectedly. After some deliberation, the package was allowed to continue on condition that the batteries were removed first this time.

THE WORST TRAINSPOTTER EVER

30-year-old Alan Witherbee is a man who takes his enthusiasm for trains too far. He was prosecuted for stripping naked by the side of a railway line in

Vermont, USA, and committing
'a lewd act' as a freight train
rolled past – much to the horror
of the train's conductor.

Police arrived at the scene
to find Witherbee now fully
clothed again and loitering
innocently by his pickup truck.
When asked what he was doing
there, Witherbee explained
that his truck had overheated
on the way back from a bar in
New York. When the officers
called the bar and found it to

be closed that day, Witherbee
came clean. He knew something
they didn't – that he had been
charged with doing something
similar just a year previously.

Witherbee avoided jail this time,
but on one condition – that he
'remain fully clothed when the
potential for public viewing exists,
with an exception for swimming.'

DUTCHMAN TAKES THE P*SS

What should you do if you have a urine fetish but not enough urine?

What you shouldn't do is sneak into the women's toilets at Rotterdam airport and arrange plastic bags under the toilet seats to catch the stuff. You'll get caught, like one Dutchman recently did.

Hauled up before the judge, the urine-harvester didn't have

much to say for himself other
than that since being busted, he
had 'learnt to satisfy himself
by watching porn instead'. For
reasons unknown to anyone living
outside Holland, this touching
story of rehabilitation persuaded
the judge to let the man off with
a two-week suspended sentence.

DUCK DOESN'T TAKE NO FOR AN ANSWER

A male Dutch duck achieved worldwide infamy recently after chasing another male into a glass window, killing it, then having sex with the corpse for an hour and a quarter in front of a crowd of bystanders.

The window belonged to the Rotterdam Natural History museum, the curator of which proceeded to write an entire scientific investigation into the world's first proven case of homosexual necrophilia among wild ducks. It didn't take the academic world by storm but it did win the curator an Ig Nobel award for the year's most useless scientific research.

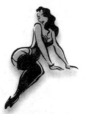

JAPANESE GROPERS FIND STRENGTH IN NUMBERS

A group of Japanese 'railway gropers' have formed the world's first pervert's union... The Chikan Tomo-no-Kai, or Gropers' Brotherhood, is an organisation devoted solely to the feeling up of women on Japan's notoriously crowded commuter trains and is said to include Buddhist priests, doctors, and civil servants.

The group holds regular training

sessions, according to an insider.

"We all pool our money and employ several girls who let us grope them while actually on the train," the groper revealed. "We do it in teams of six, and take turns on the girl while the others observe. Afterwards, we'll go to a coffee shop and critique each other's technique."

The Brotherhood meets once a month in a Tokyo bar to swap stories and techniques as well as to award each other martial arts-style belt rankings for groping proficiency. 'Black belts' are expected to touch the buttocks of 100 women a month, and one member has earned the super-rank of 7th Dan for his ability to escape pursuing police officers.

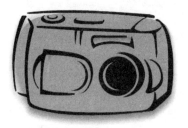

FLASH PHOTOGRAPHY

Most photographers display
their work in galleries. Jeffrey
Pritchert displayed his photos
on women's cars. Unfortunately,
Pritchert's pictures were all
of his naked genitals. Most

'viewers' reacted badly to his work and called the police.

41-year-old Pritchert, of Arizona, USA, recently admitted to leaving his work on the cars of up to 100 women over a six-year period. He was caught after a huge operation in which officers staked out car parks all over the state until they finally caught him decorating the windscreen of another victim. His most famous picture is now his mugshot.

GOAT MAN UNSURPRISINGLY 'EMBARRASSED'

A New Zealand man who admitted trying to have sex with a goat escaped jail after his lawyer told the court that he had since been given 'a hard time' by members of the public.

41-year-old George Kepa, broke into a tin shed in the town of Nelson, where he was caught 'unsuccessfully trying to have sex with the goat'.

Kepa, who already has six pages of prior convictions including one for 'indecency with an animal', was sentenced to 150 hours of community service after the judge's heart was softened by the defence's account of the 'embarrassment, shame and the hard time from certain members of the local community' that Kepa had suffered.

MAN GETS LUCKY WITH PIG

Police officers called to a disturbance at a London inner-city farm recently found the cause of the disturbance to be a 72-year-old man copulating with one of the farm's pigs.

The elderly gent was caught red-handed with his pants around his ankles by officers, who later told the press that he was fortunate to have picked a friendly pig for his muddy tryst. According to a police spokesman, any of the other pigs 'would have done him some serious damage'.

The man probably wasn't that pleased with his good luck.

AMERICA'S WORST-DRESSED CRIMINAL

A frantic police chase in a small American town ended with a cornered suspect fleeing into a supermarket, cops hard on his heels, wearing nothing but a T-shirt and a 6-string.

"I saw his ass and it wasn't cute," remarked a bystander. "He should have done some bodybuilding or something."

Police had originally wanted to talk to the man after it was realised he was driving a vehicle that had been reported stolen. After briefly giving them the slip, however, the suspect was reported in a nearby town, 'waving people over to his vehicle and exposing himself'. The chase resumed at speeds of 80 mph before police deployed a 'stinger' to burst the man's tyres, causing him to flee on foot into the clothing department of the local Wal-Mart.

"All I could hear was him saying he was sorry," another witness told the local newspaper after the fugitive had been dragged away with a towel around his waist.

THE DANGEROUS WORLD OF PANTY FETISHES

Two underwear thieves' lust for women's knickers escalated into a fight that left one of them dead. A 51-year-old Malaysian named as M Priasamy came a cropper after a violent scrap with his accomplice over how to share out a bag of stolen smalls from his neighbour's garden.

Priasamy was struck several times over the head and died

at the scene. His accomplice was arrested later and charged with murder. In a happy ending, however, the neighbour got her pants back.

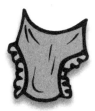

CHINA/JAPAN RELATIONS NOT HELPED BY ORGY

Tensions between old wartime enemies China and Japan still run high, especially on the September 18th anniversary of Japan's invasion. Top marks then, to the organisers of an orgy on 2004's anniversary in which 400 Japanese men were flown into the Chinese city of Zuhai to have sex with 500 local prostitutes.

The 500 prostitutes were collected

from Zuhai's surrounding areas and bussed en masse into a 5-star hotel where they 'entertained' the Japanese men for three solid days, according to reports.

The party only came to light after the men had flown home again, leaving China fuming and several of the organisers facing lengthy prison sentences for their part in what a livid government official called 'a law-breaking incident of extreme squalidness'.

BRIDEGROOM'S HAPPINESS DEFLATED

It's always difficult when a husband's parents disapprove of his wife. When the wife is a blow-up sex doll, grief is guaranteed.

A 44-year-old man from Rio de Janeiro recently introduced his folks to the blow-up doll that he claimed was his new bride. According to a friend, the man was so in love with his sex aid that he talked to

it constantly and thought
nothing of bringing it to dinner
with his religious parents.

In a story fitting of Shakespeare,
the man's 71-year-old mother
demanded that the pair be
separated. She then drove her
point home by cutting a hole in
the doll with a pair of scissors.
Outraged by his mum's rudeness,
the man strangled both of
his parents on the spot.

NO LAWYER IS THIS IMPRESSIVE

When you're on trial, the last thing you expect to happen is for the judge to start masturbating, but it can happen – as one French defendant now knows.

Witnesses at the man's trial in Angouleme Magistrates Court were disturbed to see the judge 'raise his official gown, open his trousers and perform unmistakable movements' as the man's lawyer was pleading his case.

The judge was referred for psychiatric tests. The French authorities didn't seem to have considered the possibility that it was just a really, really good speech.

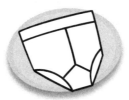

SHOE HOARDER ONLY LIKES LEFT FEET

Ichiro Irie, of southern Japan, is a very fussy shoe thief.

When women's shoes began going missing at a hospital in Southern Japan, a simple stakeout led police to Irie, who was followed and caught red-handed.

A search of his small flat revealed a whopping collection of 440 stolen shoes – all for the left foot. Astonished police waded through a mountain of high heels, leather pumps, sandals and even nurses' shoes, but couldn't find a single right-foot shoe anywhere.

When questioned, Irie could only explain that he had 'a penchant for women's feet'. His reason for his obsession with the left foot remains a mystery.

PERV ARMED ROBBER ISN'T GREEDY

Italian police are still hunting for a single-minded armed robber who held up a sex shop in the city of Milan. The man didn't seem interested in the contents of the till at the Night Shop in the city's downtown area - after waving his pistol at the shop assistant, he made off with just a blow-up sex doll and a woman's full-body leather bondage suit.

TRAFFIC CAMERA WANTS TO LIVE A LITTLE

Viewers of a boring traffic channel in Alabama got more than they bargained for recently when one of the channel's live traffic cameras began zooming in on attractive women's breasts.

Regular viewers were puzzled to see that Channel 45, which normally shows a rotation of clips from all cameras in the city of Tuscaloosa, was only showing the view from one camera which was following attractive women down the street and zooming in on their breasts, legs and buttocks.

Furious city officials launched an investigation which revealed that the culprit could have belonged to any one of these: the Tuscaloosa Department of Transport, the Alabama Department of Transport, the Tuscaloosa Police Department or the Alabama State Police – all of whom had access to the camera's controls.

AFGHAN SOLDIER MAKES AN ASS OF HIMSELF

Men in southwest Afghanistan are traditionally required to pay £3000 to the parents of the girl they wish to marry. If they're broke, they have to wait.

Sometimes the long wait can do funny things to a man. Police recently raided an abandoned house in the province of Paktia and found an off-duty soldier having sex with a donkey.

The man languished in jail for several days, expecting the worst. In a happy ending, however, policed released him after he convinced them that he'd only done it because he had no hope of affording a wife in the foreseeable future.

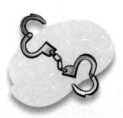

THE HAIRCUT BANDIT

Californian women with long hair can rest a little easier now that Michael Lynn Howard has been apprehended. Howard, a hair fetishist, was responsible for snipping off several women's ponytails and running away with them.

Howard, known as the Haircut Bandit, became sexually aroused specifically by the sound of scissors cutting long, dark hair.

For three weeks, he terrorised the Long Beach area with his scissors until police finally apprehended him trying to bag a woman's waist-length ponytail at a bus stop.

Police who raided his home after found hair strewn all over his flat, which contained an impressive collection of 'hair fetish' videos.

"There were videos of naked women getting their hair cut," the prosecutor recalled at

Howard's trial. "There were videos of Howard cutting women's hair, and some of a couple who had cut each other's hair and shaved each other's heads. There was a Spanish game show where they would cut your hair if you got the question wrong."

The 47-year-old Haircut Bandit pleaded guilty in court and was jailed for eight years.

A MAN IS A DOG'S WORST FRIEND

A former animal shelter worker on trial in Belgium for having sex with dogs came up with an original defence – he claimed that did it because he felt sorry for them.

Many dogs, explained the 36-year-old man, can't have sex – especially the ones locked away in animal shelters. Despite facing a jail sentence of six months, he happily admitted to having selflessly helped the dogs achieve sexual satisfaction.

There was one detail that the dogs might not be so happy about, though - it also emerged during the trial that the man had posted thousands of pictures of his canine couplings on the Internet.

PROBABLY THE BEST BOSS IN THE WORLD

When the head of a Danish IT firm found out that his workers were mostly using the company's Internet facilities to access porn, his reaction was very enlightened.

Levi Nielsen, head of LL Media, was checking up on the websites that his staff visited and found 80% of them to be sites of the 'left-handed' variety. Not wishing to risk 'cranky behaviour' by repressing the needs of his employees, he subscribed all his staff to the porn sites at a cost of £3 per employee per week.

The downside for his employees is that they are now only allowed to access their new job perk after they've done all their work for the day.

PORN LIVENS UP A DULL DAY IN PARLIAMENT

A Croatian MP, bored with a debate on road traffic safety, decided he'd rather be watching pornography instead. He didn't wait until he got home though - he simply switched on his laptop and stuck an X-rated movie into its DVD player.

"Within a few seconds, he had the attention of all his male colleagues," said a witness who maintained that no one was bothered by it. "It was very amusing," he added. No action was taken against the MP, who took in a good five minutes' worth of filth before rejoining the debate.

MEDICAL FETISHIST BANNED FROM HOSPITALS

53-year-old Norman Hutchins, a 'medical fetishist' with a thing for surgical masks and gowns, has become the first man to be banned from every National Health Service hospital in England and Wales.

A court recently heard that unemployed Hutchins harassed NHS staff for medical equipment on 47 occasions in five months. He is said to have told staff things such as 'he was playing a doctor in an amateur play' or 'he needed them for a fancy dress fun-run'. He was finally banned from all NHS premises after becoming abusive on occasion.

"NHS staff should not have to tolerate such behaviour from anybody," said a spokesman. Hutchins was eventually jailed for three years for his behaviour and branded 'a menace to anyone involved in medical or dental institutions' by the judge.

PORN NOW SAFE FOR THE RELIGIOUS

Devout Jewish Internet pornography enthusiasts can sleep a little less guiltily thanks to a rabbi who has invented a new prayer especially for them.

'Please God, help me cleanse the computer of viruses and evil photographs which disturb and ruin my work,' reads the prayer written by Rabbi Shlomo Eliahu of the Israeli town of

Safed. He devised it because he was worried that Internet sex sites were putting family relationships at risk. The rabbi recommends that web users recite it before logging on, so that they'll be spiritually covered for anything that might happen.

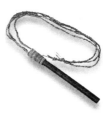

EX-COP NO LONGER TAKES PIG JOKES WELL

A former policeman from Norway has been fined the equivalent of £700 after being caught in the act with a farmer's pig.

The farmer, who noticed the man loitering near his pig pen, crept up to the pen with a camera. When he saw the ex-copper 'fondling the pigs', he began snapping.

"Suddenly he pulled his briefs down and did what I didn't think was possible," the farmer later recalled. He took nine pictures of the incident, all of which he handed over to the pig-lover's former colleagues.

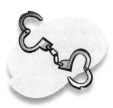

DIY SURGEON'S CAREER SNIPPED SHORT

A 29-year-old engineering student in Taiwan has become the first person ever to be prosecuted for castrating men for their own sexual pleasure.

Shou-Shan Wang, who lived in a quiet suburb in Michigan, USA, advertised his 'medical' services on an Internet group for men with a testicle-removal fetish. His 'patients' flew him all around the world to perform his operations, which he claimed to have learnt from watching his grandfather, a genuine doctor. Wang admitted to police that he'd performed the procedure on over 50 men in total.

The DIY surgeon was finally rumbled after his neighbours noticed a 48-year-old man staggering around in the street outside Wang's house. According to police, Wang had taken 40 minutes to castrate him on his kitchen table, after which the pair had sat down for dessert. The missing testicles were in Wang's fridge.

Luckily for Wang, he was only convicted of practising medicine without a licence. After all, his patients were all volunteers.

NAKED DOG-WRESTLING WOMAN 'DOES IT ALL THE TIME'

Police officers, responding to reports of screams and barking in a normally quiet American neighbourhood found a naked, middle-aged woman wrestling with a large dog in a man's garden.

Officers say that when they asked the woman what she was doing, she told them

that she was having sex with
the dog – and claimed that
she did it all the time.

The dog's owner, woken from
his slumbers, couldn't confirm
that the woman 'did it all the
time', but did recognise her.
He remembered that she was
often friendly towards the dog
when she walked past the house,
adding that she had been 'acting
strangely' in recent months.

The dog couldn't comment,

although a police spokesman later observed that 'he's obviously a friendly dog and was having fun.'

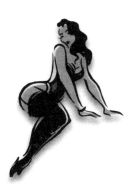

KIDNAP FANTASY FAILS TO AMUSE POLICE

A sex game led to chaos in Holland when police received a report that a woman was being kidnapped. Three men had been seen bundling the woman, who was handcuffed, gagged and blindfolded, into a van in the town of Brunssum.

20 officers were scrambled and the van was pursued by car, motorbike and helicopter

to the nearby city of Heerlen, where it was caught in a roadblock. The men were bundled out of the van at gunpoint and their victim was freed.

However, the woman began screaming at the officers who'd rescued her, calling them 'stupid bastards' and howling that she'd been 'trying to set this up for months'. The kidnap had actually been a carefully planned sex game, in which the three men were participants. All

were released without charge
after a stern telling-off.

"We advised the lady next
time to arrange to be
kidnapped in her own home,"
said a police spokesman.

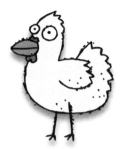

THIS IS CLUCKED UP

Life can be tough when you're a chicken. Take the story of one hen from Zambia, for example.

First of all, the chicken's 50-year-old owner attempted to

have sex with it in his house.
He wasn't successful because
the chicken squawked so noisily
that the man's wife came in to
investigate the noise. She realised
what her husband was up to and
did what any loving wife would
in such a situation – told their
entire village. Their neighbours
turned up to 'admonish' the man,
who put an end to the discussion
by killing himself in front of them.

So did the chicken receive a kind
of justice? Not really. Keen to

draw a line under the whole
episode, the villagers killed it too.

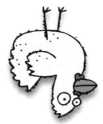

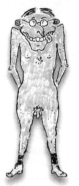

If you say a modern celebrity
is an adulterer, a pervert and a
drug addict, all it means is that
you've read his autobiography.

P.J. O'Rourke

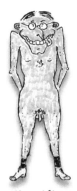

Chastity:
the most unnatural of the
sexual perversions.

Aldous Huxley

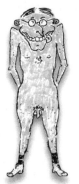

Some mornings, it's just
not worth chewing through
the leather straps.

Emo Phillips

In Conclusion

I SAT ON IT BY ACCIDENT, HONEST...

In what could well be the best magazine article ever, two American doctors have compiled a list of things that have been removed from hospital patients' rectums. Writing in Surgery Magazine, Drs. David Busch and James Starling produced an

inspirational list of examples
- a document that suggests
that the pinnacle of human
creativity can only be attained
when inserting things into one's
backside. The list includes:

32 bottles, one with a
rope attached to it.

Foodstuffs: a cucumber, an
apple, a potato, a carrot, a
whole salami and a turnip.

14 vibrators and ten sections
of broom handle.

Sporting equipment: a pool ball, a tennis ball and two baseballs.

One man had managed to insert an entire axe handle. Seven other bright sparks had light bulbs removed from their rectums.

Many cases seem to have involved cooking enthusiasts – a knife sharpener, a mortar pestle, a plastic spatula and a 'tin cup' were all reported.

Extra points for safety go to the man who managed to 'lose'

an oil can with a whole potato wedged over the sharp nozzle.

Our country cousins made a good showing – there were three separate incidents of cow-horn removal, as well as cases involving a 'frozen pig's tail' and a 'kangaroo tumour'.

A piece of wood *and* a peanut was a nice touch, as was a curling iron, a box of candles and a large bottle of shampoo.

The grand prize, however, goes

to the person who managed to get a pair of glasses, a key, a pouch of tobacco and a rolled-up magazine up there all in one go. Sir, you've made us all proud.

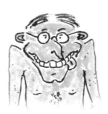

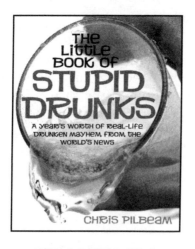

THE LITTLE BOOK OF **STUPID DRUNKS**

A YEAR'S WORTH OF REAL-LIFE DRUNKEN MAYHEM FROM THE WORLD'S NEWS

CHRIS PILBEAM

ISBN 1-905102-23-2

£2.99

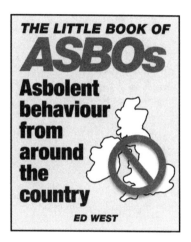

THE LITTLE BOOK OF

ASBOs

Asbolent behaviour from around the country

ED WEST

ISBN 1-905102-41-0

£2.99

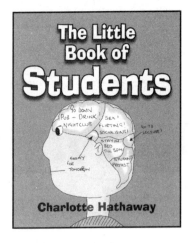

ISBN 1-905102-26-7

£2.99

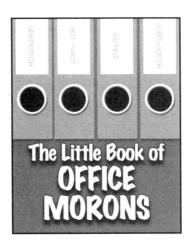

ISBN 1-905102-28-3

£2.99

Are you or a friend a perv?

Do you have any embarrassing pervy stories?

Tell us, we want to know: pervs@crombiejardine.com

All Crombie Jardine books
are available from your High
Street bookshops, Amazon,
Littlehampton Book Services, or
Bookpost (P.O.Box 29, Douglas, Isle
of Man, IM99 1BQ.
tel: 01624 677 237,
email: bookshop@enterprise.net.
Free postage and packing within the UK).

www.crombiejardine.com